5/18

W9-DFS-714

Chronic Illness
as an access to
Quantum Healing

Passing through the Eye of the Needle
into Self-Actualization

JENNY RUSH

Wilbraham Public Library
25 Crane Park Dr.
Wilbraham, MA 01095

Copyright © 2015 by Jenny Rush
All rights reserved. No part of this publication may
be reproduced without prior permission in writing
from the author.

ISBN: 978-1-4951-8233-4
Contact Jenny by visiting
www.lymethriving.com

Dedication

To my husband Dennis and our daughters, Nicole and Samantha. No words can possibly convey how grateful I am to have you as my family, and no words can express the deep pleasure of the friendship that arises from it. Thank you for loving me.

To my Mum and Dad, without you my life and this book would not be. Thank you for your timeless love and support.

"It is not in the learning of something new that we discover our true identity. It is the un-learning of that which we believe to be true that has us realize the truth of who we already are. In this realization is peace and self-empowerment for thriving with and through chronic illness."

Table of Contents

CHAPTER 1
Starting Over

As I headed down toward the river, the wheels of the mountain bike jarring over the uneven dirt road, I could feel the emotions rising in my chest. Tears began to stream down my face. Cindy was already at the river, had laid down her bike and was sitting quietly, taking in the surrounding scenery. I rode up, laying my bike next to hers and walked over to sit beside her, still crying. She turned and was immediately concerned. What was wrong? Was I starting to feel sick again?

Our friendship had begun 45 years previously, two little girls in their first day of ballet class. That day was followed by six years of being in the same classes at school and ballet, and side by side in a variety of sports teams. When I was twelve I went to boarding school. It was the beginning of an intimate, long-distance relationship that became even longer-distanced when our family moved away from South Africa to the United States. We had stayed in touch through all the years in whichever ways technology and finances allowed: letter writing, three-minute phone calls, recorded cassette tapes, emails, Skype calls, text messages, and then, even longer phone calls. We reveled in the face-to-face visits every few years, sharing our families and watching each other's children grow up, and always, sharing our hearts in love, laughter and tears as life unfolded in all its splendor.

What continued to feel so special to me in this relationship was the freedom to be myself, to be able to ask for anything and never feel like it is a burden. It was made obvious again as she picked me up to head into the bushveld together. I knew she was juggling a lot of work projects and family commitments at the time but, despite that, she arrived promptly after breakfast with the car fully-loaded with food, two mountain bikes, and all the other bits and pieces we might need for our time away. She showed up hilariously at the front door wearing a mask and snorkel; there had been severe flooding in the area we were heading to, but nothing was going to get in the way of our 'Thelma and Louise' getaway. Oh, and did I mention that my middle name is actually Thelma and hers is Louise?

This particular visit we were enjoying was precious in so many ways. It was a 50th birthday gift from my husband, Dennis. After having struggled with my health for a number of years, I arrived in South Africa enjoying my eighth consecutive day of feeling remarkably well. I had a sense that this trip, to the country of my birth, would represent my life starting over again. There had been no interruption in this delicious experience of wellness almost two weeks later.

So there we were, in January of 2012, on the border of the Kruger National Park, resting next to the river, surrounded by the sounds of hippos and birds, and I was weeping. It was difficult to translate my feelings and experience into words for Cindy, but words tumbled out anyway. My sense of wellness and wellbeing was so profound that it literally felt as though I'd never been ill before, ever. It had been a week of taking walks, riding bikes and game spotting. We ate our dinners under a night sky so clear we could see the Milky Way, all the while enjoying brief visits from nervous warthogs. After spending the better part of the previous year lying on the couch, it felt completely miraculous. I was overflowing with gratitude and wonder and love. Cindy listened quietly as my tears and words gushed out, and she sat quietly as I quietened, and she bore witness to my life starting over on the banks of the Crocodile River, in the country where I had been born.

Feeling so deeply humbled by this profound sense of renewal was in large part due to the revelations that were the result of my experience of illness the last year. It hadn't been the only year of illness, but it was only in that last year that I had fully surrendered and allowed the gifts of the illness to reveal themselves.

This is the story of my awakening; the unfolding of self-realization and true healing. It was not about learning anything new or finding something to believe in. It was a process of un-learning what I had previously believed to be true, a year of letting go that ultimately revealed the truth of who I am and who we all are. It had left me deeply grateful for an illness I thought might end my life or perhaps remain a constant in it. This was not about being grateful for the circumstances of struggle, but rather for the experiences provoked by the struggle that when investigated, revealed the blockages to true self-expression and to the knowing of who we are.

As part of a large community of people suffering with chronic Lyme disease, I am committed to making a difference to any and all. To borrow a phrase from Marianne Williamson: "I share (my lessons) with an open heart, I hope you will listen with an open mind."

CHAPTER 2
A Pattern of Illness

Lyme disease was the diagnosis, somewhere around 2001. The symptoms had been easy to overlook initially. I had a hectic schedule and was busy with our two young daughters. It was no stretch to believe that aching elbows and joints were the result of over-training in the gym or that the tiredness was just typical of moms like myself with young children. The fatigue and pain had become progressively debilitating over the course of a year, so I had booked an appointment with a rheumatologist. He ran a variety of blood tests checking for lupus, rheumatoid arthritis, Lyme disease and other illnesses. The wait for the test results seemed an eternity, so when the phone rang I was relieved. I eagerly listened to the nurse as she shared that I was positive for Lyme disease. To be perfectly honest, I was thrilled with the diagnosis because I had been harboring a deep dread that the tests would reveal rheumatoid arthritis. My busy and athletic life, driven by a rigid mindset, had no room for curbing any physical activities. A few weeks of antibiotics would take care of everything and life would return to normal--or so I thought.

Six months later I was pulled off the fifth different antibiotic being used for treatment, IV Rocephin, because once again I had begun having an allergic reaction to a drug. I felt significantly worse than when I had begun treatments, so it was with relief that the catheter was removed. Somewhere inside me was a breath of hope that all the treatments had done some good, and that as soon as I cleared my system of residual drugs I would experience the benefits and begin to feel better. I couldn't get to the health food store fast enough, and once there I purchased a juicer and a bag full of organic vegetables. Although I had no experience with juicing, my gut instinct told me this was the next step.

Two months later I was feeling well enough to begin my morning runs again. I was out of shape by that point, but over the weeks I regained my fitness and slipped easily back into life as usual. Over the next seven or so years I had occasional bouts of deep fatigue. The familiarity of it had me wondering if it was Lyme again, but after a few days it would dissipate and I'd forget about it and go on with life.

I did not know anyone dealing with Lyme disease, I didn't know much about the disease itself and wasn't aware that it could be chronic. However, with my newly revealed sensitivities to antibiotics, I *was* aware that a recurrence of Lyme disease would mean facing a complete unknown. Without any knowledge of chronic or recurring cases of Lyme, however, I wasn't particularly worried.

By the end of 2008 it started again: deep fatigue and a general sense of malaise. And as before, it took a while before I went to be tested. My schedule was significantly more demanding than it had been in 2001. I pummeled through the days, frequently on 4 hours of sleep with a large travel mug of coffee in hand. Having gone through a rigorous leadership training program for 6 months, I was now enjoying being a coach for participants in the next program, and shuttling myself between my home in Connecticut and New York City felt worth the effort to revel in the deep satisfaction of this newly revealed passion. At the same time I was running a small business, the children were in high school, and getting to the gym was routine. The leadership coaching activities consumed almost as many hours as all the other activities combined. But it was the fatigue that was the clue. Debilitating fatigue goes so far beyond being extremely tired, and I've only ever experienced it during Lyme disease. The tests were positive again. I didn't know how fortunate I was to have a positive test result, since I had no idea that the standard Lyme tests are notoriously inaccurate.

An open-minded and compassionate medical doctor, knowing of my sensitivity to antibiotics, referred me to a bio-resonance practitioner who administered the treatment sessions and put me onto an herbal protocol. He was very knowledgeable about Lyme disease, having had his own personal 18-year experience with it. The progression back to wellness was gradual and gentle, and after several months I was feeling almost normal again. I hadn't paid much attention to the dietary recommendations but had really enjoyed the meditation sessions that were run concurrently with the bio-resonance. As soon as it felt like I had my feet underneath me again I was back to my busy life as usual. And then I started to feel sick again....wash, rinse, repeat a couple more times.

Up to this point I had never found a tick on me, nor had I seen a bull's-eye rash.

Late in the summer of 2010 we took a family vacation to Spain. While we were there I noticed a red mark on the back of my thigh that looked like an insect bite. It didn't itch, but it grew slowly bigger as the days went by. My thought was that it must have been a spider bite. I looked forward to getting back home the next week and putting some over-the-counter medication on it. Within a few weeks it was covering half the back of my

13

leg and creeping around the front of my thigh. Never did it occur to me that it was a tick bite, especially since I was back to feeling quite well. And then it turned purple, the glands in my groin swelled up and I eventually ended up in the emergency room with cellulitis. The kind ER doctor said she would be testing me for Lyme and other tick-borne illnesses, despite me being adamant that it wasn't Lyme disease, because I felt well. I was treated in the ER with an IV antibiotic for the cellulitis and put on 2 weeks of doxycycline. I was sensitive to the medication but could tolerate it. A week later my test results came back positive for Lyme and Ehrlichia. I felt unwell on the antibiotics, but once I'd finished them and a week or two had passed, I was feeling pretty normal, and so, as before, I went back to life as usual.

By December I was beginning to feel sick again, and by January I was so ill I had withdrawn from most of my commitments. This time it was different. This time the experience of illness lasted a full year, this time there were many days I felt I was fighting to live, this time there were weeks I didn't want to live, this time I un-learned things I believed to be true, and this time I experienced *true healing*.

The year began with a realization. There was a momentary flash of seeing my life from a broader perspective, like seeing the forest and not just a tree; illness was a repeating pattern in my life (MY life) and with that realization came the tickle of knowing that uncovering the source of the pattern would empower me and interrupt it. And so began my journey through the eye of the needle.

CHAPTER 3
Acceptance

To accept is to receive what is offered or given. Life deals us all sorts of experiences, including illness. We always have the choice of accepting or resisting what comes our way. Accepting illness does not mean that we have to like it or that we are not willing to do something about it, but resisting that it's there or pushing against it doesn't make it go away either. Accepting that we are immersed in an illness experience is simply being with the truth of what already is. Acceptance allows for peace.

There is nothing wrong with dreaming about what we wish for. In fact, creating positive images or thoughts about what we do want, and aligning or identifying ourselves authentically with them causes a shift in our way of being and in our experience of life. When we do not make peace with where we are in the moment, we remain acutely aware of what we do not want and the gap between where we are and where we feel we need to be creates a great deal of suffering.

Acceptance didn't come readily to me. It was disappointing to feel myself being dragged back onto the couch. I was accustomed to an overly busy life, one that included intense physical activity. After spending a large percentage of my life as a competitive athlete, I had enjoyed withdrawing from competitive events like triathlons and bodybuilding to engage in endurance activities like kayaking, biking and occasional mountain climbing. What I hadn't noticed was that I continued to train exactly the same way, pounding my body in the gym as though preparing for a competition. It somehow seemed necessary to be fighting fit at all times so that I could pick an endurance activity to participate in, any activity, without much notice. Somewhere in this long history of sport I had begun to think of myself *as* an athlete, not someone who simply enjoyed sport. It had become an ingrained part of my identity. I had not been aware of how my identity was given by all the things I did, so along with losing my identity as an athlete, I was also losing my identity as a small business owner, and had been failing to show up in any typical way in all other areas of my life too.

I struggled deeply with not being fully available to our daughters. Nicole's high school years had vanished in a blur and she was now away at university in Colorado. Somehow through the haze of my seemingly rudderless life I helped her move into her new home, feeling sure I was missing so much of her excitement in my every-present need to just crawl into bed, away from all stimulation. She blossomed in the adventures of her new life and committed herself to her studies, suddenly showing up as an independent woman. Where had I been? Samantha was in high school, and for what seemed like an eternity, was a flash of comings and goings from the house as she dealt with her teen life. The guilt of not reaching out to her was smothered by a superficial relief that she appeared not to want parental guidance. I felt I had nothing to offer. There was a turnaround moment when she sat by my side on the sofa and asked me about how I was feeling. She listened without getting hooked into my stories and I noticed she had matured into a graceful young woman. How had that happened without a mother?

My attention turned away from the life I was accustomed to as I busied myself with treatment protocols. I slowly but surely began connecting with other Lyme patients on Facebook. The previous year someone had kindly reached out to me and offered the support of a Lyme group, but it hadn't appealed to me at the time. There was a well-entrenched conversation in my mind that I didn't need anyone's help, so I was surprised to eventually find myself pleased to meet Lyme patients in online groups.

It was comforting to know that I wasn't alone in my daily struggles and rituals, but I was completely shocked to hear that some had been ill for years with debilitating symptoms, some for decades, and so began my education about chronic Lyme disease. When it came to information about tests, medications, alternative treatments and physiology, the group members often sounded like scientists. I felt like a complete kindergartner. Different types of groups had been formed, each offering something unique; groups for people treating with alternative methods, groups for people in specific geographic locations, groups for parents of sick children (mostly the parent(s) were sick too) and so on.

We firmly believed in fighting against the illness. We would not accept it. We were determined to live, although there were times the determination dissolved into depression and despondency. It was distressing to discover the frequency of suicide deaths in this community and I had no idea that there would come a point in time when I too would face that level of apathy in my own journey.

Being aware of how many struggled desperately with insomnia, I felt fortunate that most nights I slept quite well. But it was disheartening to open my eyes after seven hours of sleep into a fatigue so deep I wasn't sure I had the energy to make it from the bed to the bathroom. Tears would often sting my eyes as my spine was called

17

upon to make its first movement of the day. A night of lying still made my spine rigid, as though it had been transformed from bones and soft tissue into wood. Making the first movement of the morning required that the wood be 'shattered' to allow for flexibility. I knew that once I was moving around it would ease, but I dreaded the morning's explosion of sensations. The day would follow with strictly regimented protocols. There were other normal details of life to tend to, as well as commitments in my small business, which thankfully wasn't requiring too much attention at that time. Other than that, I was on the couch.

It was early in 2011 and a two-day seminar I had signed up for the previous year was drawing closer. I wasn't sure whether I should attend, or even if I would be able to attend, but I was sure it would support me in some way. It was a pilot course and the topic was described as, 'the neuroscience of the brain, its natural programming to survive, and ways to shift ourselves out of the realm of survival and into a space where we are free to create our lives in a way that fulfills us through the things in life that are important to us.' I made the decision to participate and informed the course leader that I was struggling with cognitive issues, amongst other things, and that I would leave if I felt too ill to continue participating. He smiled reassuringly and said it was not a problem.

And so for two days I sat like a zombie in my chair, missing bits and pieces of conversations and working through the exercises. Sometimes I cried with the effort it required to participate, but ultimately I was able to get the gist of it. The benefit was astonishing: I uncovered acceptance.

Going into the course I felt that I had lost my life to Lyme disease. Very little of my life resembled its previous form, but stumbling out of the course a couple of days later, everything felt different. I had the realization that in fact I DID have a life, and it was the very one I had, and it *included* Lyme disease. Life looked different to how I thought it should look before I entered the course, but over the weekend we had explored life without the 'shoulds,' and without them I saw life was simply what it was, as it was, and it *was* my life. There was something for me to deal with physiologically around the illness, and I was committed to being proactive with my protocols. Not only that, but I had a say in how the illness experience was occurring to me and how I was choosing to respond to it. In other words, I didn't *have* to feel like a victim and I was free to choose how I would experience and use this life challenge. Stepping into a place of freedom of choice reduced the significance and indignation of my victimhood.

During the course I had distinguished that some of the things important to me in my life were: making a difference for others, learning to honor myself, and personal growth, and I recognized that I still had an opportunity to make that a reality even though it would look different to how I had previously imagined it. New pathways immediately became visible, new possibilities for my life became real. In other words, even with illness, I could still fulfill things important to me in my life, and Lyme disease could actually be an access to that. I had a newfound passion to be a Lyme activist, and this could satisfy my need to make a difference for others. Addressing my physiology with an appropriate diet, comprehensive protocols and learning to rest could address new ways of honoring myself, and continuing to delve into a personal inquiry could fuel my personal growth.

And there was a quietness right alongside the exuberance, and life was good, and Lyme disease was a part of it, despite the fact that my body and brain still felt like hell.

But old habits die hard. I found myself revisiting old ways of being that were still very ingrained in my thought processes. One such thought process (belief) was that I *should* always be productive in some way. Unbeknownst to me, being productive was one of my ways of continually trying to prove my self-worth.

There was a day when, lying on the couch, I was surprised to find myself feeling quite peaceful and slightly well. I was not paying attention to my thoughts and so my patterned way of being kicked in: "If I feel good then I should get up and do something...I *should* be productive." I rolled off the couch and attempted to get something done. I started by working to clear my email inbox, but my brain jumbled the words of each sentence and the task seemed monumental. I attempted to complete a work project (web site development), but the request from my client required mental gymnastics to decipher, putting my brain into overload with the feeling that it was about to short-circuit. The fatigue hit me like a massive gray cloud, my limbs felt heavy and my brain was only able to operate in super-slow motion. I dropped myself back onto the couch only to find that, about 10 minutes later, I felt quite good again.

Contemplating that experience triggered a memory of something I had learned in my previous coaching activities: to make a difference for a person struggling with an issue, we meet them where they are, listening to them without judgment or our version of their solution. In so doing, they feel heard or validated, and can then take their attention off their particular story and their need to be heard, which then creates a clearing in which their next step in addressing their issue can be revealed to themselves, by themselves.

With this remembering I turned back to my current experience and applied it. The pieces began to fall together and I had the visceral experience of being heard and validated by myself. Where I was in the moment was not well. When I met myself there and honored it, I simply lay on the couch with a resulting experience of feeling content and relatively well. As soon as I began to get busy doing things, no matter how simple, I experienced the gap between what my body and brain were capable of and what I was demanding or expecting my body to do. In that gap was the wishing for something that wasn't, the yearnings for the past and the empty hopes for the future. It was my suffering.

Upon further contemplation I become aware of how I had not met myself where I was at, ever. In the past I had barreled through, stepped over, forced myself to DO what I felt *should* be done, rather than just be with myself exactly where I was, without the need for justification. I had just uncovered a patterned way of being (doing, doing, doing), informed by a belief (being productive proves self-worth), that until then had been hidden from my view. From its formerly secret place it had been an exhausting motivator. With it now fully in the light, I had the option of making a different choice. I could choose to be productive, or I could choose to rest. Neither was right and neither was wrong. Whatever my choice, there would be a result that was directly correlated to it. And for the first time, it would be because I chose it, and being free to choose is empowering.

And so each day I had this opportunity to accept and meet myself where I was, to honor my body and my mind in the quiet for which it had been yearning. This was a new experience for me. I practiced it repeatedly. The practice evolved and transformed and I discovered for the first time what it felt like to honor myself in this one small way. I was surprised by how nourishing an experience it was and I felt the roots of my Self grow a little deeper.

It really felt as though gaining some understanding about acceptance, and then implementing a way of being that was accepting, was facilitating the release of a blockage in the flow of life. This beautiful experience of flow felt like a rush of freedom. However, it also brought to the surface of my experience the next blockage to address. It was as though I had had a glimpse of the forest again, but was now back with my nose against a tree.

I was headed from the kitchen to the living room where my trusty couch awaited. It was a typical day that brought a myriad of physical symptoms and fatigue. Once again I had accepted my state of ill health and knew that lying down was needed and appropriate. But something was beginning to gnaw at me. I 'turned' to investigate the feeling. It was guilt. With my attention fully on it, I quickly discovered that there was quite the narrative that came along with the guilt. It seemed quite effortless to list the reasons that guilt was appropriate. I wasn't doing much of anything except tending to myself. Dennis was covering the mounting expenses. He was also managing most of the parenting duties, traveling extensively for work, and tending to the minutiae that I used to address. I tried not to talk too much about what was going on with my illness, but when I began struggling cognitively, I broke down in tears and told him. I feared that my brain function might decline to the point where I was like an Alzheimer's patient and I had to let him know. Another time I came across a clinic out of state that seemed like a possible option to check into for some intensive therapy, and I mentioned this to him as well. Without hesitation he said that we would do whatever needed to be done. My heart just cried rivers in gratitude and guilt, as this occurred to me as an unfair financial burden. All in all, I just felt like such a burden. As is his rock-steady and generous nature, he somehow juggled everything without complaining. Despite that I still saw the overwhelming impact on him in the chaos of his office and the stress in his face. I didn't get to the source of the guilt at that time, but I was fully aware of it, and somehow I was able to accept that this was just where I was, and trusted that over time it would be resolved. In the meantime, even in the face of the guilt, I continued to do what I felt was best for myself.

This lesson around acceptance was not 'handled' and out of the way. It was simply available to implement whenever I chose it, but sometimes when a different challenge arose it seemed I had forgotten it altogether. I soon discovered that each new understanding or lesson can be broadened and deepened for as long as we draw breath. It also seemed that I was just at the very beginning of retraining my brain's default way of performing.

CHAPTER 4
Surrender

There is a difference between acceptance and surrender. As an analogy, imagine that somebody has given you a blue sweater. When you receive it and keep it, you have accepted the gift. It isn't particularly relevant whether you like it or not. With no obligation to keep it, you place the sweater on a shelf with your other sweaters, perhaps never wearing it, but you have accepted it. Surrendering would be wearing the sweater and allowing yourself to experience what it has to offer, such as how you feel or look wearing the color blue, or discovering the sensation of the fabric against your skin and the warmth it does or does not provide. Surrender isn't about our thoughts; it is about being fully open to experience.

Surrendering is not actually an 'act' or a 'doing,' it is what occurs when activity of the mind ceases to have our attention. It is when that which we have been resisting is allowed. It is not a process, it is the present moment exactly as it is. However, it can be followed by a process of deepening our understanding of how and why we avoid being fully present.

At the peak of illness, I found myself once again in full resistance. It was a day like many before: the fog in my brain swirled endlessly, my head felt twice its normal size and weight. Every joint in my body wept and my spine ached as I waded through the sludge of deep fatigue. Every corner of my body seemed broken and I felt like I was dying. With tunnel vision focus I resorted again to aiming all my energy on not dying. At that time I was dragging myself to five appointments each week, visiting two different chiropractors, receiving bio-resonance treatments, having an occasional gentle massage, and seeing my naturopath. In between the appointments and sleeping, I was taking a large amount of supplements, juicing fruits and vegetables, detoxing, and filtering gallons of water to drink. I stubbornly held onto drinking a glass of wine (or two) in the evenings...something may as well have been enjoyable. And all the time I was repeating in my mind, "I will not die, I will not die."

With my sorely challenged brain I followed the lead of other Lyme patients, researching fanatically, unable to mentally retrieve all I had read, but continuing my research anyway. I was determined to stay alive.

I had begun to post questions in the Facebook groups and was learning new information. Sometimes I was receiving support, sometimes I was offering it. That always felt good, the giving and receiving. I was continually shocked to newly learn about what other people were dealing with, and I became even more committed to shedding light on this overlooked community and disease.

But on that one day, my brain that felt so withered away released a quote I'd heard a hundred times before, "What you resist persists." I was stunned! How had I not seen what I was doing? I had gone back to living in a complete state of resistance and I was completely exhausted from the effort.

And so in a fit of exhaustion and with the electric prod of that quote I stopped trying to figure everything out, I stopped trying to not be sick, I stopped trying to control my life, and I flopped onto the couch. My biggest fear was of dying, but in that moment I accepted completely that, like everyone else on the planet, I would die, and I accepted the possibility that I could die from this illness. I lay there without thoughts about anything. It was full surrender.

I stared at the ceiling. I was aware of it but had no thoughts about it. There were cobwebs in the corner. I was aware of them but had no thoughts about them. I looked through the glass sliding doors and saw the trees. I was aware of them but had no thoughts about them either. I became aware of simply being aware. I became aware that I had always been aware of being aware, even if I had not noticed before. As I lay there being awareness itself I knew, with a knowing beyond my mind, that the awareness had no beginning and no ending, that it is completely still, and that it is peace itself. I was knowingly aware that this awareness was the "I" that I had spent my life referring to without being present to the reality of it. I was aware that this "I" was not my body or mind. And I was aware that the "I" that I am is the one same "I" that everyone is. There was some image behind my mind that revealed the sameness that we are, the interconnectedness of this "I" expression into our reality, that we are all of this awareness that is the ISness that is. But the image can't be shared or described. It is beyond the limits of language or mind. In surrender I knew the Oneness we are and the richness that is life, and that our fullness and completeness is experienced in the gap between words and the pause between actions.

Quietly I became aware of my mind again. Somehow it seemed to gently translate this knowing into experience. The first thing I experienced was a relief that was extraordinary. Until that moment I had had no idea how much energy I had been investing in resistance or expending on being who I thought I was or should be.

The words "just be yourself" suddenly made sense. There was the immediate knowing of how effortless it is to simply be our natural self-expression without referring to others' opinions or our own judgments. It is the allowing of what already is.

The second thing I experienced, with absolute certainty, was that "I," not Jenny the body/mind, but "I" my true Self, was not broken, had never been broken, and could never die. And I was aware that my body was dealing with something. To be identified with that which is aware of the body, that which is already whole and complete, provides a steadiness that is not affected by the changes in life.

The third thing I was surprised by was that, despite a great deal of reading and seeking through a variety of teachers, the actual moment of self-realization required no knowledge, no action and no teacher. It was the most effortless moment in my life. It was simply being who I already was. The overriding experience in the moment was of profound, unconditional love, of being whole and complete, and I was completely fulfilled. It was the first moment in my life when I needed absolutely nothing.

Most of my life's activities had some expectation of the fulfillment of those experiences. Being a parent, being in relationships, running a business, having dogs, participating in sport, traveling....each of these could provide the sought after experiences all humans long for: peace, love, happiness, fulfillment. But there I lay, the fullness of all those desired feelings, completely inactive, completely alone, and desperately ill. In a single moment of self-realization there was nothing I needed from an outside source or created experience. It was the ultimate liberation.

My mind disentangled itself from the energy drain of resistance and fear, leaving an empty space in which peace expressed itself into my experience. I was at peace with how I had lived my life, at peace with possibly leaving our two daughters without a mom, at peace with my successes and failures, at peace with my humanity. I cried quietly, not with sadness, but with relief and love. Perhaps it was simply an outpouring of forgiveness for myself. I knew without question that regardless of any circumstances that life could offer, I had access to total fulfillment and peace. Everything in my body, down to the smallest cell and beyond, relaxed out of fight or flight into expansiveness and peace.

I had certainty going forward that I was free to strive for what I wanted, knowing that if I failed I still had access to whatever would have been provided by the objects of my desires. It felt so different from creating a future that was derived from need. To create out of need solidifies an attachment to an outcome, which then immediately limits us through the fear of failing.

This moment of surrender left my life forever altered. It was the ring of a bell that can never be un-rung. It was the release of all things, thoughts, feelings, and perceptions, and the slipping through the eye of the needle into the no-thingness of consciousness. But being fully identified as the awareness or consciousness we are was not how I had lived the previous 50 years of my life. There were and still are patterned ways of being that are not aligned with my true Self, and as I went forward they started to reveal themselves, one by one, tugging me back through the eye of the needle in reverse into this very real experience of being a mind and body in a universe of matter. And so began the deepening of my understanding and the accepting that I would never be done with this introspective work.

29

CHAPTER 5
Self-Responsibility

Self-responsibility, as a way of being, empowers you to be fully accountable for your own life, for your thoughts, for your body and for the way you experience life's many ups and downs.

No matter what challenges life presents, it is always possible to be self-responsible in the moment. Being self-responsible is not about being a failure or being blamed for something, it is simply a place to stand that allows us to be empowered in the face of those circumstances, regardless of what they are, and it IS a choice. There is no requirement to be self-responsible and it is not wrong to choose to experience any aspect of life from the position of victim. But from time to time I remembered the realization I had about illness being a pattern in my life, as well as my intention to get to the source of it. I was clear that investigating anything and everything that felt like it was a blockage to the flow in my life would contribute to revealing its source. Without question, feeling like a victim was a blockage.

In the case of Lyme disease, I found it easy and natural to believe that I was sick due to the bite of an infected deer tick. It was definitely not my fault. I was gathering more and more information to validate my position of being a victim. It wasn't difficult. There was information that proved the 'incurability' of chronic Lyme, that proved a large population of the medical profession didn't believe the chronicity of the illness, that proved the lack of support from the governing medical body and insurance companies, to say nothing of the CDC that affirmed those positions and contested opposing points of views by other groups of Lyme literate physicians. In exploring that position on my illness, I noticed that I was choosing to be a victim, and this just didn't work for me. Victim, as a way of being, was not providing anything to support healing, forward movement or self-empowerment. Anytime I rested back in all the evidence I had gathered, I was nailing my foot to the floor as I waited for someone to 'save' me, to change treatment guidelines, to come up with a cure and to relieve me of any responsibility in the matter of my health.

The turnaround came slowly but surely. My primary care physician was Dr. Gary Gruber. He patiently shared information, explaining how the immune system works, the impact of leaky gut syndrome on the function of the brain, and the integration of body, mind and spirit. My naturopath talked and I listened. On my brain's worst days, he sounded like the adults in Charlie Brown--"Wah, wah, wah." And somehow, what he shared was being stored away for when I was ready to remember and deal with the information. And not only was he a great source of scientific information, he also provided a space I simply healed in. I'm not referring to healing in the physical realm as much as the emotional realm, although physical healing was underway even when it didn't seem obvious. There was no judgment. He listened to what I was dealing with, accepting my decisions to add to his protocols, giving me feedback on my choices, all to empower me in my journey. This was generosity. This was someone committed to my wellness. It was the Naturopathic Physician's Oath in action.

From my place on the couch and in the quietness of doing nothing, Dr. Gruber's words eventually made their way into my consciousness for contemplation. I felt my ego mind stand up and say a few choice words! My ego, so desperate to win, to be right and hold me hostage as a victim was not happy. A deeper awareness of the ego mind had begun to arise during times of self-investigation. My understanding was beginning to deepen as it became clearer that the ego played an important role in survival. But somehow its blanket response to so much of life was only serving to validate its self-importance, way beyond what was actually useful. I was becoming aware of how nourished my ego felt when there was internal agreement with its righteousness and indignation, and at the same time, noticing the impact of that in my experience of life. Being dictated to by my ego always served to cement a sense of separation, of being 'better than' or 'less than,' of being a victim, and letting go of this provided the opposite in humbleness, connectedness and love. But I had newly experienced surrender and I was not looking to lay blame.

It unfolded and revealed itself: The human body is designed to heal itself. It is an environment, one that we contribute to with our thoughts, feelings, beliefs, foods we eat, hours we rest, exercise we undertake, toxins we absorb, ingest or inhale, professions we enjoy or don't, stress we feel, joy we share and so on. I was not sick because a bacteria-infected tick had bitten me; that was simply the tipping point. I was sick because by the time the bacteria was introduced into my body, my immune system was so off balance that it was unable to fight the bacterial invasion.

And then a question arose, "Who is responsible for my immune system, for the state of my wellbeing and the level of wellness existing in MY body?" Clearly it was my responsibility.

This realization did not land in my consciousness in a way that made me feel wrong or at fault; it simply landed and planted instant roots. I couldn't shake it off and, to be perfectly honest, didn't want to. It was a 'Wow Moment': I had created my life just as it was! I had laid the foundation *myself*.

I'd already tried on the victim outfit, and let me tell you, I wore it well. I cried because I had 'lost' my life, was afraid, was very ill, and I felt sorry for myself. And rightly so, I might add: the disease was no picnic and my life had been dramatically altered. And then a question surfaced, "So, how's this working for you, this being a victim?" Let's see.... Uh, not so well.

And so I wore the self-responsible outfit each day, examining the seams, the buttons, and the experience I had in it. What a difference! The whining and ceaseless chatter in my mind went quiet. The scenery of my life was no longer through the image of a tick and various spirochetes. Now it was *my* life again, and there was something to be responsible for, the rebuilding of my immune system and creating myself as an environment that did not support the proliferation of the Lyme bacteria. It was such a delicious experience, finally shifting from being a victim to being in charge of doing what was necessary to restore the integrity of my immune system.

I leaned on experts in various natural healing modalities to support me, but they were no longer responsible for my body. I was responsible, and I was responsible for choosing the team to support me. It was around this time that I started to explore how I had tended to illness in the past. Always, it had been me going to a professional to fix me. It had been about killing off what shouldn't be there. Until my experience with Lyme there had always been a medication to handle this. Now I was faced with learning to trust my body and its ability to heal, and to accept its current position of being out of balance as well as its tendency to restore a healthy balance. My body was like a building, the foundation of which had settled unevenly, causing cracks in the walls. We addressed the cracks to make my body as comfortable as possible, but the real work was leveling the foundation, my immune system. I was the foreman on this reconstruction project, and I gladly sub-contracted out to other professionals.

Being a perfectly imperfect human being, there were periods of time when I stepped back into the victim role and did some serious whining. I think I might even have raised whining to a high art form. Those periods of whining eventually shortened. There was less satisfaction or juice to fuel my ego mind as I became quicker at identifying when I was playing the victim. I might even have had moments of compassion for myself, forgiving a very human response to a trying situation.

Of course, I had many questions to contemplate. What had I been doing to compromise my immune system? What was the flavor of my thoughts over my lifetime? How did I manage stress? How had I depleted my rest cycles? And of course, why? There were so many questions to ponder. For the moment I just rested in this new experience of self-responsibility. In due course I would begin to address those questions and the answers would unfold at just the right moment.

CHAPTER 6
Context is Decisive

We can powerfully alter the experience of our illness and what we discover about ourselves as a result of it, by simply shifting our context around it. The opportunity for addressing context came up when my dear friend, Cindy, called me out on my repeating complaint of, "I hate swallowing pills."

I was standing in the kitchen, a huge glass of water in hand and pills lined up on the counter. "I hate swallowing pills"--gulp/swallow--"I hate swallowing pills"--gulp/swallow. My daily routine revolved around the many supplements I was taking daily, and I complained bitterly to her.

"And if you are hating each pill," Cindy asked, "how effective do you think they will be for your body, given that energy follows thought?"

That abruptly stopped me in my very negative thought track. The context was negative and disempowering, and if energy did follow thought, I wondered how the energy of those recurring thoughts might be contributing to stalling my body's healing process. I truly didn't enjoy swallowing pills, but since I was committed to taking them, it seemed highly worthwhile to make each pill count.

I thought about this for a while, knowing that I was free to create any context I wanted, and I was clear that whatever the context, I wanted it to contribute toward my healing. I made a decision to shift my context to *kindness.* Each pill I swallowed was going to be an act of kindness toward my body and my immune system. I didn't have to suddenly begin liking the pills, I just had to put my attention on this new context. At that particular point in time I was swallowing about 80 supplements per day, so I had the opportunity to be 'kind' to my body that many times per day.

With each pill I swallowed I imagined my body receiving and celebrating the introduction of additional vitamins, minerals and enzymes, putting all of them to use wherever their sustenance was required to fuel repairing and rebalancing. It didn't feel kind right away, but I did notice the radical difference of this way of thinking about these daily activities. By the end of the first week it was noticeably easier to focus on kindness, and the effort to remember to activate it lessened. Two weeks after beginning this practice, something happened. I took a handful of supplements with no thought. I wasn't even aware that I had forgotten to create a context of kindness in the moment. What had captured my full attention was the experience I was having; the visceral feeling of warmth all around and through me. I wanted to fold my arms around myself so that it couldn't escape. I walked slowly down the hall to the couch, lay down and floated in it. It was so beautiful, so soft, so kind, so new. And then the realization came forward: this was the experience of being kind to myself, an actual, real experience, created by me, experienced by me. I wanted to know why it felt so new. I searched my life in an effort to reveal previous experiences of kindness. There were many. But what I couldn't find was any moment in my past where I had provided this for myself. Not one.

It was as though someone had turned on a bright light, bringing previously shadowed parts of my life into full view. With my inherited athletic genes I had thoroughly enjoyed competing in many sports, for decades, training hard but rarely nourishing or resting my body appropriately. There was no kindness, just demands upon demands and expectations of performance. It was becoming clear how I had not been grateful for, or been kind to, a body that had been worked so hard for so long. And somewhere inside me was the tickle of newly knowing how I had contributed to the current state of my ill health. It didn't occur as a failure, just as an innocent ignorance. In the deep humbling of this realization came an understanding that it would take an extended effort to restore the balance in my body that I had spent decades undermining. Somehow I was content with not knowing how long that might be, whether months, years or matching decades. It just felt good to know that each action I took to nourish and replenish my immune system was one step closer to repaying a debt.

This newly uncovered access to experiencing kindness was soft and gentle, and despite my physical symptoms, was now available on demand when I authentically aligned with kinder thoughts.

This was not the first time that the exploration of context had come up. Without fully appreciating it at the time, wellness as a context had been introduced to me by my two chiropractors. The care they provided was inside of a wellness model rather than a sickness model. I had the opportunity to be steeped in a wellness education and to shift the context I had around health care. It was a focus on promoting the body's ability to heal itself, just as my naturopath had been doing. And while I was very enthusiastic about this wellness model that resonated so deeply with me, there is a difference between knowing something well and actually putting that knowledge into practice under one's own steam. And so, with my new experiential knowing of how shifting my context could alter the way I experienced life, I explored creating a wellness context for myself during my illness.

Putting my illness into a wellness context sounds illogical, but I did so anyway. In examining it, my illness experience showed up somewhere on the wellness spectrum, some days closer to the high end, some days closer to the low end...but either way, I was able to view it as a level of *wellness*. If I was floundering in the lower end of the spectrum there were things I knew to do to improve my 'rating,' or at the very least, contribute to the possibility of improving it. It supported me to keep my attention on health rather than on sickness. With a focus on what I wanted I was automatically drawn to health related articles, inspiring documentaries and empowering conversations. This often shifted my mood to inspiration. However, there were days I still subjected myself to a sickness context. I would think and talk about myself as being sick and feeling broken, all of which was a negative label or interpretation of what was simply the expression of my body. The difference was that at least I was aware that I had created that context and subsequent experience, and I realized it was simply a choice. Being aware of making a choice, without judging it, was automatically empowering.

Bringing the illness experience into a wellness context shifted another of my thought processes. Perhaps it was more of a realization as a result of the wellness context. In my mind's eye I saw my body as a group of systems, all working together. For instance, if there was inflammation in my joints it was expressed as pain. If my body was dealing with leaky gut syndrome, there was the noticeable expression of brain fog. The actual expression was not a judgment or point of view from my body. It was simply expressing the exact balance of all my systems, without the label of sickness. It was pure expression. It seemed quite beautiful to know that these uncomfortable experiences were a result of my body functioning exactly as it was designed to. It was quite a revelation to know that sickness was a label assigned by my thoughts about what my body was expressing.

As the weeks and months passed I became more practiced at noticing what I was doing and thinking, reminding myself to create context that worked to keep me moving forward and feeling in charge. I noticed along the way that it was a real challenge when one symptom or another was highly activated. The true color of my context was always revealed when my feathers were ruffled. That's when I reaped the benefit of having people around who hold me accountable for my life experience. While this was sometimes, to be perfectly honest, incredibly annoying to my ego self, ultimately they are the best friends I have. They pushed me back onto my own two feet, leaving it up to me as to whether I created wellness, kindness and self-responsibility for myself or not. And the choice was always mine.

CHAPTER 7
Surprise Gifts

During illness I didn't particularly look forward to taking the dogs for their morning walks. The mental and physical effort required to get moving often seemed insurmountable, but this was a case when an ingrained and routine way of doing things served me well. Trail walks were simply something we did almost every day, fulfilling on my promise to provide Ben and Thandi a good, healthy life. I wasn't oblivious to the benefits it provided for me, but it was challenging when I was ill, so occasionally we would skip a day. And so, as was my morning routine, I rolled out of bed and began to get dressed. They know exactly what clothes I wear when we are headed for the trails. A pair of jeans means no walk, ratty sweats and thick socks means, "TRAIL WALK-- WOO HOO!" That cold and snowy morning had them gleefully watching me as I dressed in layers of clothes. I walked slowly down the stairs holding onto the banister as the dogs barreled past me in a rush of anticipation and joy. My joints and spine grumbled with the first movements of the morning. I drank a green smoothie and took my first batch of supplements.

And so off for my morning dose of dog therapy I went. They led by example, enjoying every new scent, expressing joy for the outing as though it was an unexpected gift. And my therapy session began.

I noticed the quiet of the air, the whiteness of the snow and the crunching sound of my boots as I broke through areas where the surface of the snow had softened and then refrozen with the fluctuating temperatures of day and night. I looked for evidence of what they had their noses glued to, seeing only tracks where they smelled a past presence. The cold air rushed in as I unzipped my jacket to cool off my rapidly heating body and the freshness was delicious. I became present to the stillness within me, uncluttered by thoughts.

But the peace receded suddenly as a rush of thoughts flooded in: Had I forgotten to do something yesterday? What did I need to get done today? What was on the grocery list and when should I go to the store? Would I get any work done? How is my friend feeling? And on, and on, and on...

A sudden tangle of leashes jerked me back into the present moment. I noticed that I had left the dog therapy session, giving it up for thoughts that were mostly about things past and future, about things that didn't even exist in the moment. Those few moments of losing presence had felt so busy.

And so we resumed the session, slowly navigating over fallen trees and rock piles, breathing heavily from the exertion, enjoying the morning quiet of the woods and the company of each other.

This was a gift from my dogs: the peace of presence. They taught, by example, that life is rich, no matter the length of the to-do list or the circumstances of my life. My daily dog therapy provided an opportunity for me to start each day following their example. I practiced bringing the quiet presence of those walks into my daily life, aware that this was yet another underdeveloped muscle that would eventually begin to respond to the repetition.

The months went by slowly until the early signs of Spring became apparent. The daffodils were offering a tiny splash of green in an otherwise gray landscape, and the bitterness of the winter cold was being moved aside with a gentle surge of warmer air. My winter coat, boots and gloves were happily left at home for less encumbered trail walks in sneakers and light fleece jackets. My body was still offering a plethora of physical symptoms and I felt sure that the couch was beginning to conform to the shape of my body.

On an unseasonably warm and especially beautiful late spring morning, something remarkable happened. As we returned home from one of our walks I became aware of an absence of symptoms. What was this? Ben and Thandi jumped out the car and we went inside. Still no symptoms. Really, what *was* this?? I began taking inventory of myself. My brain felt clear, my joints felt lubricated, and my energy level felt normal. Everything was neutral. So now what? I went back to the garage and looked at my kayak. The weather couldn't have been more perfect to go paddling! There was a flurry of thoughts about whether this feeling of normalcy would remain or evaporate, and if it did evaporate, when might that happen? In this brand new experience there was nothing I could refer to that satisfied the addiction of my mind to knowing the answer.

I put my dog therapy lessons to work. I would simply stay present in each moment and honor what it revealed. It played out with me hauling the kayak onto the roof of the car, strapping it on, throwing my life vest and paddle on the back seat, and then stopping for a moment. I took inventory of my body after the exertion. Everything felt normal, so on to the next step. Thirty minutes later I was parked at my launching spot on Calf Pasture Beach in Norwalk. Another inventory...the drive

45

hadn't depleted me. I unloaded the boat and equipment. Inventory again...and so I took each step, committed to reversing them should I feel a sudden shift physiologically. Once I was out on the water, paddling toward the islands, I just let go. I put a halt to the inventory checks and surrendered to the experience of the moment. What pleasure! The sun was warm and the water received each dip of my paddle with a gentle splash. The red hull of my kayak glided through the liquid offering of the Long Island Sound, and 30 minutes later I was sitting in total astonishment on the sandy beach of my favorite island. Being a weekday, there were no other boats around, and so I inhaled the beauty and the quiet and swam in gratitude for this surprise gift.

A few hours later I was home again. I couldn't help myself; I took an inventory. Truly, I was blown away. I still felt completely normal.

A day later I was fully back into the illness experience. I wasn't surprised or even disappointed, my attention was fully on this remarkable reprieve I had just lived through, and the true gift of it eventually made its way forward past the circumstances of that glorious day. I knew, without a shadow of a doubt, that the expression of wellness was within me. And I knew, without a shadow of a doubt, that what remained to be done was to continue to remove the blockages to its full expression. Wellness had not been taken away from me by an illness, it had been covered over. Once again, despite the overwhelming physical sensations of illness, my sense of wellbeing was soaring in liberation and humility.

CHAPTER 8
Grieving

"Warrior: a person who shows or has shown great vigor, courage, or aggressiveness."

A point of inquiry had arrived where I was contemplating "Warrior." It wasn't uncommon to read words of encouragement in the Lyme community that included statements like, "Stay strong Lyme Warriors! You can do it!" Aren't we all warriors at certain times in our lives? When we are fiercely committed to something we engage in the corresponding actions with vigor and tenacity. And even if we temporarily lose our footing on the path, our commitment has the warrior in us fight our way back with renewed enthusiasm and commitment.

For a variety of reasons I used to enjoy thinking of myself as a warrior. For one, I was aware that typically when I really put my mind to something, I would achieve it. Perhaps it was part of my personality, or perhaps it was just a way of being that had been well developed over the years during sports practices. But I don't remember referring to practice sessions as 'practice.' For me it was always 'training,' a quirk I was unaware of until one day I was asked, "What are you training for?" This question was posed in response to me explaining my unavailability for an event because I would be in the gym 'training.' I was a bit taken aback in noticing this, and offered a rambling reply that I preferred to be ready to respond to any sudden desire to launch myself into an endurance activity.

But most likely, right next to knowing with some amount of certainty that I would achieve a goal, was my ego enjoying being all fluffed up and special: "Look at me, I'm winning--I *am* good enough." I was okay with knowing this about myself. It's part of being human. It would only be later that I truly benefited from recognizing that particular conversation of my ego. But at that point in time my focus was on the warrior I had known myself to be, but had now seemed to have lost.

I was giving everything I had to addressing my illness, tending to my body, doing what I could to relieve myself from the exhaustive symptoms of fatigue and pain, and exploring my emotional barriers. I wasn't doing it perfectly, but I was doing it warrior-well. However, no matter how much ground I had gained along the warrior's path back to wellness, there were times I simply put down all my warrior weapons and cried.

On one such day I had been rereading some of my blog postings and it had given me some snapshots of where I had been earlier that year in comparison to where I was in that moment. A great deal of ground had been covered and the progress seemed noteworthy. And yet, in an attempt to restore one simple activity back into my life (a half-hour gym workout twice a week) I found myself back on my knees with a slow brain and a flare-up of symptoms. The emotions that arose with this were deep.

With each lesson that had been revealed I found myself catapulted forward into a space of gratitude, and then hungrily, greedily, pushed forward for the next expansion and another fix of spiritual liberation. I was being a spiritual junkie. Despite thinking of myself as a spiritual being having a human experience, I saw how I often forgot to honor the human experience. And I was, after all, here for the human experience.

Surveying my life in that moment I saw a quietness I didn't have before, peacefulness with less frenetic activity, and a love of self that was growing. I was learning to simply BE.

And yet there was a life I once had that was vastly different, one in which I could rush around and do whatever I chose: over-achieve, over-do, over-spend, over-eat, over-drink, under-sleep, and over-train. It was fun and it was stressful and it was out-of-balance. I was not sorry it was over, and yet I felt a deep loss.

It was as though I'd lost a close friend, one who was not always good to me but who had always been there, through the good times and the bad. I had let her go without regret. I knew that she created an unsustainable way of living and that I was currently addressing the results of that, but now, I simply missed her.

With my wellness-warrior face set aside, I cried as I mourned the loss. I grieved every part of the life I had once known; the 'me' I'd thought I was, the jobs, the friendships, the activities, the late nights of socializing, the dreams, and the ignorances and naiveties. This grieving was not only normal, it was a healthy letting go of the past.

Some friendships survive only a finite period of time, serving a purpose, and then it is time to let go and move on. Some days I struggled to let go of the person I used to be, afraid she would be forgotten somehow. But knowing that in time she might be forgotten was comforted by a certainty that she would always be loved. My warrior-heart told me this.

CHAPTER 9
Lighten Up

Standing alone in the kitchen one Sunday morning I found myself crying again. My body and brain felt awful. Looking over at the counter covered in bottles of various enzymes, vitamins, minerals, herbal remedies and more, I sighed. I couldn't face going through the daily routine of pills, detoxes, making green smoothies or forcing my brain to do the dance of comprehending simple things, all the while fighting my way through the heaviness of fatigue.

So I discarded the looming protocols and looked at the large, homemade chocolate chip cookie in my hand. With a glance over at the 'torture counter' I decided, "Screw it, I'm eating the cookie, and I will eat junk and comfort food all day."

And so I ate the cookie, still crying.

Five minutes later I was counting out my pills, organizing myself to make smoothies and filtering water. I was glad I had allowed myself a start to the day that felt so dramatic. Sometimes it was just how I felt: all dramatic and sorry for myself. I was certainly tired of the slog through Lyme, and that Sunday was not a good day for sure. I had been to Whole Foods to stock up on detox stuff and on my way out answered a survey at a table by the exit door. A woman asked me a series of questions. I couldn't decipher what she was saying, my brain was jumbling everything up, but the funny thing was that I was answering her, and I had no idea what I was saying. I probably left her as dazed and confused as myself.

But that bad morning, with a moment of lightening up, morphed into a reasonable day as I filled up on things good for me. Doing things that were good for me was still a fairly new experience. Not only that, but I was doing them at a slow pace. At almost 50 years of age I had not spent many of those years being good to my body. I tended to learn the hard way, but it's okay, I do eventually learn. I sometimes worried that in this case, I had learned too late.

I hated and loved dealing with this illness. In previous rounds of Lyme I thought I had tended to myself with gusto. But there is a remarkably different level of tending when you feel like you are dying. I am far from perfect, and sometimes found myself face-first in the dirt, not taking care of myself, but the scale was tipping. It was my full-time job to manage my care. And for the first time in my life, I wished I had someone to hand it over to.

My life had become simpler in a way. At times there were the deep pleasures of doing simple things like laundry or taking the dogs for a slow walk. I even drove below the speed limit, something I found quite amusing. It had become necessary because my brain couldn't process information at a normal speed, and would quickly go into a panic when over-stimulated. I was quite astonished as I became aware of how much information we are continually processing.

I shared a chuckle with friends when I recounted a trip to Boston Market. I was craving chicken with all sorts of additives and seasonings not typical of my diet. I had ordered a whole chicken, all white meat, and then in all seriousness requested that they cut the chicken up.

I bemusedly told of how I had to write myself sticky note reminders so that I could remember simple tasks requested of me, only to discover later, when asked about them, that not only had I not completed them, but I had little recollection of writing the notes in the first place. For some reason I found it slightly amusing to notice the absence of stress when it came to to-do-lists, because I had no memory of the lists' existence. I wondered if it was like that for some Alzheimer's patients.

I had gone from being the ultimate 'doer' to someone who spent a lot of time sitting in silence, just being. That was often all I could do. And in the quiet, I experienced life in a different way. I couldn't quite articulate it, perhaps because there weren't words to describe the exquisite intricacies of life, or perhaps there was a fog between my experience and my outward expression of it. At the time there was just a mass of experience and new knowing that existed within me. I was aware of a growing passion and purpose for making a difference with chronically ill people. Little pieces were falling into place. In the meantime, as I took stock and healed, I spent my quiet time staring at the ceiling from my customary place on the couch, knowing that part of me was burning with aliveness, and it was exactly as it was meant to be. I was aware that this aliveness was not being expressed outwardly. One of my daughters had made a comment in passing that I seemed to be so far away. I tried to assure her that I was totally fine on the inside, and that my body was in some way working to catch up, but I'm not sure I communicated it very well.

There was an inkling of knowing that the moment I stopped wishing for life to be any other way was the moment I would have learned what there was for me to learn from this lesson, and I would be done with Lyme.

And then it would be on to the next lesson, during which time I would probably find myself saying, "Screw it, I'm eating the cookie."

CHAPTER 10
Depression, an Access to Love

"Roller coasters go up, roller coasters go down. Apparently I picked the mother of all roller coasters to ride. The past few weeks have been a series of whiplash ups and downs. Today I'm at the bottom, in the pit that feels never ending, but that is reliably followed by an up. Onto this certainty, I hang with fingernails.

I was standing in the kitchen earlier, crying--yup, must be Sunday. Another inventory-taking moment. Pain that is making me twitch, stiffness in my neck, fatigue. I don't want to be here, I feel too tired to make a smoothie and don't much care anyway. However, I took supplements and had a cup of tea. My friends all have their own things to deal with and I'm tired of complaining about my stuff to them.

So, this is the bottom, again...feeling helpless, alone, sorry for myself, unwell... depressed."

I had begun that blog posting about falling into depression, but had stopped, unable to write anymore. I had read and reread the words and was struck by how I was being about this experience. I didn't know what I hated more, the experience of feeling like a victim, or stepping back and observing how I was *being* when I was feeling like a victim. I knew this was simply not who I was at my core, but I have to say, sometimes I allowed this ass-kicking experience of illness to get the best of me.

I had been ramping up my protocols until I was taking or doing something to support my body every 90 minutes, from 9 AM until 9 PM, day in and day out. The time was approaching for a fresh round of blood tests and so, as instructed, I went off all supplements for about five days. Much to my surprise, I felt absolutely great for several days in a row. It was almost a shock. My body let go of its fluid retention in three days (eight pounds of it), and I felt clear and well. Without my normal 'job,' I quite honestly didn't know what to do with myself. Just as my before-Lyme life had ended, so too had my current life ended. By the end of that week I was in a pit of depression, something I hadn't anticipated in my wildest dreams.

I just couldn't believe it. After all the realizations, after all the 'aha!' moments, after knowing with every fiber of my being that I was perfect, whole and complete, how could I possibly be in this position? The peace, wonder and gratitude I had been dancing with slipped away. Had I been mistaken in what I had uncovered about the essence of who I am? Because there I was, floundering in misery and apathy.

I had experienced short bouts of depression previously, something I had accepted as normal given the nature of chronic illness, but this was different. The biggest disappointment of the day was waking up. Mostly it was starting the day in bed, crying, followed by standing in the kitchen crying, feeling empty and hollow. Time seemed to slow down in the cruelest of ways, making each miserable minute feel like an hour. There were no conversations I wanted to have, no people I wanted to bump into. The self-imposed isolation of depression was taking over my life. To start the day at ground zero felt soul destroying.

And then there was that surprising little something that would allow me to take the next step in the day, that one thing I could force myself to do next, or felt I had to do next. For me it was taking the dogs for a walk. With an unfathomable love, they would bounce into the dark mood of my room and jump onto the bed. Ben always lay on my left and Thandi on my right. Ben would put his huge fluffy paws on my chest, Thandi would put hers on my arm, and they'd look straight into my eyes with a pleading enthusiasm, sometimes licking my face for good measure. They were totally committed to the walk and to me getting out of bed to accommodate it. I was grateful for their company and endless enthusiasm, for never being put off by my depression or lack of interest in life. They loved me just as I was, no matter what, and they shadowed me as I dragged my gloomy self from one room to the next or along a trail, and all the while I just wanted to get back home and crawl into bed again.

The day usually improved somewhat. I don't know if it was because I managed to get a few things done or if because by the end of the day I could let myself stop doing things. Maybe it's because I knew that soon I could escape into sleep...no longer left with my thoughts and questions of: What's wrong with me? Will this ever end? Should I make it end? How will I make it end? I spent so much time thinking about 'How will I make it end?'

And so the weeks dragged by, each minute feeling longer than the last. It was the longest month of my life. I was waiting for some miracle that would make life worth living another day. It didn't happen.

I decided to attended a Lyme seminar, partly because attending the event would help pass the time, partly because it might help interrupt my depressive

57

thought loops, but also because I knew that a couple of my online friends would be attending and I had hopes of this bringing some small moment of pleasure into my day. I was also secretly intending to listen for some magic bullet to be revealed that would save me from myself.

It felt good to talk to people involved with Lyme in a variety of ways, it felt good to hear a doctor talk about the effects of Lyme in a way that validated my experience. But what got my attention most was the talk by an author of a book called *Coping with Lyme*. As an expert on Post-Traumatic Stress Disorder (PTSD), Denise Lang walked us through causes and symptoms of PTSD. I was surprised to learn that many chronic Lyme patients share these symptoms, one of which is severe and debilitating depression.

I did not feel I had PTSD, but it was with intense relief that I discovered I was not alone in dealing with such a severe emotional backlash from feeling chronically sick, that it was a normal part of the journey. Allowing myself to just consider that depression was a *part* of the journey made it clear that there was light at the end of the tunnel. Just distinguishing this helped me enormously.

I still began the next day lying in bed crying, I still walked the dogs. What was different on that day was that I began talking about feeling and being depressed, only to find that many of my fellow friends were in the same boat.

My mom flew to Connecticut to spend a few days with me. She appeared a bit alarmed by how thin I was but she sat on the couch near me and provided what only moms can offer--the warmth of a mother. It was so comforting.

I reached out to my naturopath. He seemed unperturbed by what I shared. I noticed that my ego mind had something to say about that. It really wanted an emotional response, it wanted the drama to be expanded on. But Dr. Gruber held firmly in a quiet, accepting and loving place. He explained that I had two components to deal with. One was the physiological cause of depression and the other was the underlying spiritual and emotional aspect. He felt confident about what was potentially causing the physiological expression of depression, but ran some tests to check my hormone levels anyway. The test results provided the information he needed to prescribe particular supplements to address the issue, and my body responded very promptly and in just a few days I felt the cloud begin to lift. But we had also had a conversation about the spiritual and emotional aspects of depression. He invited me to investigate for myself and address what was bothering me.

Knowing where to begin with this inquiry was a mystery to me, so I began a conversation with myself.

A series of surprising questions and answers followed:

Q: "What do you want most?"

A: "I want a magical person to be by my side 24 hours a day, steeping every cell in my body with a love so deep it makes life worth living."

Q: "Would this make you happy?"

A: "Yes!"

Q: "What if this person was hit by a truck and killed, then what?"

A: "Then I would be back to square one." *Sigh*

Q: "So what do you *really* want?"

A: "I want a sustainable access to the experience of love."

Q: "Since anyone or anything outside of yourself can be lost or taken away, where might you find a source that is readily available and can never be lost or taken away?"

A: "Oh, wow! The only thing that I know to be ever present in every moment of my life is me. It has to be sourced from me. I have not been looking to myself as the source of love."

It felt as though I'd just lost my innocence, that moment of realization when you so want things to be different but know in your bones that they can't be. It was the truth, and there was no way I could disguise it or pretend that it wasn't. It almost hurt as I let go the illusion. I felt so childlike and so vulnerable, almost lonely, knowing I couldn't count on anyone but myself for 100 percent reliability. But standing in the truth is unshakable, and I was aware of this. I thought back on the moment of awakening to my true Self, looking to see how it was that despite such absolute clarity I had bumped up against this childish dream.

Over time I began to realize that my self-actualization had not come as the end result of a journey during which I'd tended to myself in ever-nourishing ways, finally blossoming into the knowing. In fact it had almost gone in the opposite direction. There had been an almost accidental escape from illusion into truth, and what followed was a light shining on various stories and beliefs that were still a part of my programming, my default ways of being. It was as though I had purchased a new home but it had come with old furniture in it. My process was akin to removing the old furniture so that I could enjoy my new home. I just hadn't realized how much furniture was hidden in the various rooms until I tripped over it.

The gift of the depression was not yet fully opened. I was still pondering over why I hadn't been providing myself with the experience of love. And so the investigation continued, looking in all my dark places, noticing where I felt most confronted. And there was definitely something that was provoking me. It was like having a button on my chest that was being repeatedly pushed. My response to each button push was defensiveness and anger and indignation, and it was pushed with even the smallest of actions. Something as simple as an email or text message not replied to could surface a noticeable emotional response. I felt compelled to point out and change the behavior of anyone who evoked this reaction. I wanted *them* to stop pushing the button. A knowing eventually floated to the surface. If there was no button to push, nobody would be pushing it. I was reminded that we cannot change other people, we cannot control how someone is going to show up in life.

The only thing we have any control over is how we respond to life and other people.

By this time I was willing to address this button that I was guarding. It wasn't because I was courageous or insightful. I was simply exhausted from the futile efforts on which I was expending my energy. I was clear that the energy needed to be spent on myself.

And so what followed was one question and one answer:

Q: "What are you feeling when your button is pushed?"

A: "I feel like I don't matter."

And the floodgates of understanding opened. In a moment I was clear that my reactive experience of feeling like I didn't matter was only possible if it was a belief I'd been harboring that I didn't want revealed. I was aware that I had been side-stepping the experience of feeling like I didn't matter by covering it up with anger. Had I not had this belief about myself there would have been nothing to avoid. I might have felt disappointed at the communication breakdown, but it wouldn't have been interpreted by me to mean anything about myself. What I had been doing all my life was keeping this belief hidden, firstly from myself (because it had seemed too painful to feel), and secondly from others because I didn't want anyone to know that I was not good enough.

As I distinguished this hidden belief about myself I actually laughed out loud. This was followed immediately with a mental image of a deck of cards, each one representing a decision in my life, and as I mentally flicked through the pack I saw how every single card was shaded with the color of 'I don't matter.' With this image was the knowing that this belief was the result of a very young version of myself having misinterpreted an experience or series of experiences, and the survival mechanism that kicked in was to make sure nobody knew this false belief about myself. This played out in my life as being driven to achieve, to tend to others' needs but not my own, and to continuously prove my self-worth. My belief had been my slave master.

It was so obvious now how I was able to maintain the insanity of my schedule for so many years. My belief had been the driver of my life, it had fueled me to get to the gym on vastly inadequate sleep, it had prompted me to say yes to commitments that would take my life out of balance, and it had prevented me from making changes to my life that would restore a healthy balance.

And the understanding deepened. I saw that this was normal human behavior. It was not unique to me. It wasn't wrong and it wasn't a failure. I found myself swimming in an ocean of compassion for our humanity. My heart was simply bursting at the seams.

I turned my attention back to myself, to this belief I'd been carrying around on my back as an unseen burden or like wearing a pair of sunglasses that had colored my view of life. I wasn't sure which analogy fit best, but either way, it had been present for most of my life. This was such an expansive feeling of liberation!

I realized that in years past I might have thought of this like a 'wound,' a part of myself that remained unhealed after an experience I simply couldn't cope with on an emotional level. However, I now saw it for what it was. I was aware there were experiences that had been misinterpreted by me to ultimately formulate this belief about myself, and they were totally understandable for a child. But those events were long forgotten. What had remained of them were my thoughts--'*my*' being the operative word. AND, they were *not* true. What I was releasing was a child's *story*. There was no actual wound to heal; however, the experience of revealing this belief felt deeply healing.

The impact of a trauma in anyone's life is a very real experience, but in looking for the actual wound of it we uncover that the ongoing suffering is not the originating experience(s), but rather the result of our interpretation of that experience(s) and what we believe it means about oneself. How can we not have compassion for such innocent self-inflicted suffering that runs rampant through all humanity?

There has been some retrospective contemplation as to what prevented me from actually taking my life. It wasn't the love I had for people in my life, although I was clear how much I loved them, and it wasn't concerns about the emotional impact on surviving family members, although I was aware of the potential devastation. At my darkest point my desire to 'exit' was purely to make the unbearable feeling of emptiness go away. The apathy I felt and the bleakness I perceived were far more prominent that anything else in my experience. Being at a Lyme conference and hearing that depression wasn't unusual for chronically ill patients was the turning point. It was when I began to share what I was dealing with and finally reached out for help that had negated the need to take action.

CHAPTER 11
Lessons Everywhere

Freshly released from the tyranny of a deep-seated belief, I had a new view of life as various pieces of the puzzle began locking together. I became more and more present to the opportunities in every moment of the day, in every reaction, every doubt, every choice. In a renewed state of relaxation I reviewed some of the gifts of the journey through illness, discovering with joy that there were more than I had ever noticed.

Through the reformulating of my diet and with nutritional education, I learned that my body works hard and deserves to be nourished. I also learned that I do not have to do everything perfectly.

Through taking herbal protocols, which included the tedious counting out of many drops of remedies into a small glass of water, twice a day, over an extended period of time, I learned to commit to a long protocol, even when I did not want to, and it developed my 'commitment muscle.'

Through exploring and sometimes implementing new, self-prescribed protocols, I became aware of a variety of ways to address a similar set of issues. I learned that there is more than one way to skin a cat and we just have to find what resonates and works for ourselves. I chuckled to myself as I recalled a quote by Esther Hicks, "There are many ways to skin a cat, and any way you do it, the cat's not going to like it." In the case of addressing chronic illness, that registered as resoundingly true.

Through all the detoxing activities, I learned that if I want to bring something new into a space, I must first clear out what is already there. I applied that to wellness. If I wanted wellness to show up in my body, first I had to clear out the existing toxins, which included toxic thoughts and feelings.

Through complementary health care, like chiropractic, I learned that, just like taking my car for regular services, my body also deserves regular, ongoing care as well.

Through resting on the couch, I learned that my body deserved to rest after about 40 years of being hammered by sport, long hours of working and years of being sick. It was just time to recuperate...no justifications necessary.

Through finally submitting to being supported by others, I learned that love is present everywhere, we need only be open to it.

Even with an ever-growing list of surprise lessons, what excited me even more was discovering that quite often, doing something counter-intuitive provided extraordinary opportunities. I was becoming more familiar with my programming and belief systems. I was starting to get it in my bones that turning toward that which I was attempting to avoid almost always brought about liberation from a previously unnoticed anchor. Catching and stopping myself in runaway thoughts was giving me a small gap in which to distinguish if I was interpreting an experience, making something up and pretending it was the truth, or passing judgment on myself or someone else. I wasn't masterful at this, but as I developed this muscle of distinguishing, my sense of self-empowerment grew.

There was not one lesson that couldn't be applied to some other area of life.

Even more delicious was the exquisiteness of being more identified with my true Self. The more my false identity fell away, the more of what had previously upset or confronted me was dissolved into compassion. The sense of wellbeing felt like roots spreading out far and wide, leaving me far less impacted by changes in the weather of life. It was startling to recognize that losing my previously created identity left me fully present to nothing (no-thing), which was actually my true identity.

But there remained symptoms of illness, despite all the wellbeing. Opposing the observation of symptoms was my gut instinct telling me that the systems within my body were actually back in balance. Although I had no test results to prove this, and had absolutely no desire to submit myself to one more blood test, I remained certain of it. I resumed my investigations, feeling certain that my body remaining symptomatic was tied to my emotions and another lesson to be learned or belief to be un-learned.

In those last six weeks of exploration the final blockages to wellness were distinguished while going for energy healing and chakra balancing sessions with Bernadette. I was looking for any reason I might 'want' to be sick--or, put another way, if there was any possible 'payoff' for remaining ill. I also inquired into what I might be fearful of.

Secretly, despite all the struggles with not being able to live a normal life, I had discovered that I really, really, REALLY enjoyed resting. As soon as I admitted this to myself I remembered an annual private prayer I offered to whomever might be listening. It went something like this, "Please can I just be sick for one day, with a slight fever, so that I can enjoy lying in bed for a whole day without feeling guilty." Somewhere along the journey of my life I had decided that I had to be sick in order to rest. Well, didn't that just take the cake!

I contemplated the fear aspect and imagined what it would be like to be well and resuming an illness-free life. The emotion of it came right up. I was afraid to be well again with potentially facing the disappointment of a relapse. I was afraid of disappointment. I also knew that I was not the same person as before, and I had no idea what life would look like or how it would unfold with the 'new' me at the helm. I was afraid of the unknown. It really wasn't difficult to move forward once I saw what was in the way. As Dr. Gruber said, "Fear is an ancient mechanism of the human ego. Identifying with the fear by projecting it onto something else (disease, politics, economics, family, etc.) is the way we feel powerful, and we love feeling powerful. Yet power doesn't come from the ego, it comes from Divinity. Become aware of the fear and accept it as the survival mechanism. Let it go. Love that which is aware of the experience."

And so I let it go. My requirement around rest took a little more effort, so I created an affirmation on my cell phone that I read frequently: "You do not have to be sick to rest." That was an incredibly awesome piece of un-learning that I cherish to this day. I often take time out to rest, simply for the pleasure of resting.

CHAPTER 12
Wellness

As I noticed my familiar symptoms, I didn't wonder why I wasn't feeling well. I just knew with every fiber of my being that I had completed the Lyme journey. There was no reason to be sick, my body had been saturated in nourishment, thoroughly cleansed and rested. My immune system had been rebalanced. I had shed a great deal of emotional baggage and had come to know the essence of who I am. Nothing had been done perfectly, but I knew that perfection wasn't required and certainly wasn't attainable.

On January 5, 2012, I posted to Facebook,

"There's something between me and being completely well...and it's something I created...hidden by an [invisibility] cloak...I'm researching a visibility spell."

On January 6 I posted,

"I am well, well, WELL!"--And I consciously chose it...

On January 12 I posted,

"...What I had created that [kept] me from being sustainably well was fear...yup...gotta love the workings of our sordid little brains!"

On January 13 I posted,

"Day 7 of being and feeling well."

On January 14 I posted,

An image of the South African countryside with text across it: "Heading home to where it all began, then coming back to start again."

The next day I departed for South Africa not knowing if the long flight would interrupt my newly released expression of wellness, and I wasn't concerned if it did.

Being in South Africa was better than I could have imagined. There was a week's worth of days spent reconnecting with family and old friends, catching up on life and enjoying the pleasures of eating favorite foods and relishing the warm, dry climate of Johannesburg.

But what was pulling at me most was the desire to get out into the bushveld with Cindy, to be immersed in the scent of the long grass and the red earth. But getting away provided so much more. We were near the border of Mozambique where there had been good rains and some recent flooding. The vegetation was lush and green, the air was very warm and slightly humid.

Cindy and I were in a thatch roofed cottage away from civilization with no land phone, Internet or TV...leaving me very thankful for my iPhone with which I shared photos of each day's animal sighting with my friends and family. Our days unfolded naturally as we went for morning walks, relaxed game-spotting drives, dusty bike rides, and then exhaling the day's activities by the river at sunset.

We had not been disappointed on our game drives. We enjoyed the simple pleasure of watching Africa's wild animals in silence as they grazed or strolled through the tall grass. We listened to the songs of various birds, with Cindy identifying which they were.

And there was the ebb and flow of conversation between two girls who had enjoyed a friendship that spanned decades. Perhaps we were now women? It just didn't feel that way. I remember at one point looking at Cindy and realizing that the 'I' that knew her now felt exactly the same as the 'I' that had known her when I was five years old. It was the deep knowing of the awareness we are, every steady, never changing, no matter how life plays out.

We emptied our thoughts and experiences, we slept when we were tired, ate when we were hungry (and sometimes when we weren't) and made room for what there was to enjoy in the present moment: the awareness of the sights and sounds of the bushveld that replenished us at a soul level.

Most of the time I smelled like bug spray and my skin was sticky. The water that ran into the bathtub was light brown but amazingly refreshing. I even engaged in a midnight battle with a very large and ugly flying bug, eventually capturing it in a saucepan and releasing outside. The entire experience was sweet and nourishing.

As our friend Nandi said, "The bushveld empties the mind and replenishes the soul." No truer words could be spoken.

It was on January 26th that Cindy and I were sitting on the banks of the Crocodile River as my life started over. Nothing of my past and nothing of my imagined future was occupying my thoughts. It was the exquisiteness of being fully present in the now.

Being free from previously distinguished beliefs and stories, being aware of being aware, and experiencing life from a different perspective is difficult to share in words. There simply isn't a vocabulary that can describe what it actually feels like. The best words I can utilize are peace, stillness, expansiveness and love. But it was deeper than feeling any of those descriptions, it was actually *being* them.

With an emptied mind I was aware how each of us, at our source, are perfect love, whole and complete. Our expression of that perfection is inhibited only by thoughts; our stories about ourselves, our fears, and our beliefs. Nothing can alter who we are and always have been at our core. Our physical experience facilitates a perfect opportunity to unlearn and surrender to the true nature of who we actually are. We have everything we need within us, and our access to it is stillness. Everything is simple, although granted, not always easy.

I realized we do not have to love ourselves to be who we are. That would be like the ocean needing to add water to itself to be an ocean. It simply IS the ocean. Who we are IS love. There is simply being that expression. It is an expansive energy, it is healing, it is wellbeing, it is peace.

And so as I received myself and the Oneness we all are, I wept with the experience of a love so profound it had no beginning and no ending, and it felt like my chest would simply burst open. I reveled in the bliss of complete wellbeing and wellness. I didn't realize that my journey through the eye of the needle was not yet complete. But the beauty in the vistas from my clearer perspective were overwhelmingly beautiful, and I was deeply grateful for life just as it was.

CHAPTER 13
Flaring Symptoms...Where the Wild Things Are

Driving home to Connecticut from the airport was a visual whiplash. The long plane ride had been filled with memories of the South African countryside. I could almost smell it. But there I was in the rush of New York traffic and most of what I saw was cement. I welcomed the sight of trees in my home state as they stood proudly in winter nakedness and I looked forward to seeing Dennis. My thoughts were devoid of anything illness related.

Settling back into normal life was lovely. The trip to South Africa had released residual energies from the lessons of the previous year, and embracing life with clarity was wonderful. It didn't take long before I had a full calendar and was engaged in work projects. The most pleasurable aspect of life was enjoying it with Dennis. Without the filters of hidden beliefs it felt as though I was meeting him for the first time. Our history was not forgotten, but the energy of it evaporated in a forgiven past that now remained only as part of a beautiful texture in a tapestry that was our life together. In a new realm of relationship we looked only forward and the pleasure was indescribable. I sometimes thought we had transcended our past relationship, leaving it all behind. But the true nature of this new realm of relationship was fully inclusive. I was aware of the richness and depth of our life, every moment of our past, the good and the bad, contributing to the current moment. There is such freedom in relationship when the partners are not required to be the Band-Aid of life's old perceived wounds or the providers of happiness. It breaks any sense of bondage and the fullness of liberation brings an exquisite intimacy.

Five months later I noticed a number of symptoms that were uncomfortable in their familiarity: fatigue, brain fog, niggling pain and stiffness. The frequency of these reminders had my ego flexing all its muscles. It looked something like "roaring its terrible roars and gnashing its terrible teeth and rolling its terrible eyes and showing its terrible claws,"[1] leaving me feeling irritable and as though somehow I had failed.

From lessons I had learned the previous year I was back in self-surveillance mode. What was there for me to be responsible for? What had worked for me when I was experiencing radiant health and wellbeing that I had recently let go of, leaving me dancing with the creatures that felt like the symptoms of my ill health in years before?

The biggest change was my level of activity. In the sheer joy of living I had allowed myself to be catapulted into a busy-ness that left little to no down time. I had been dancing furiously against the clock and calendar, creating deadlines and projects. My body was simply roaring for quiet time and a schedule that included rest and relaxation.

So in the rumpus of this contemplation I burned off the frantic energy of panic and fear and was reminded of the discoveries of when I experienced the richness of life that was so fully present in the spaces between

---

[1] Maurice Sendak, *Where the Wild Things Are*.

thoughts and activities. It was all as it ever had been...perfect, whole and complete.

But I had noticed where my thoughts went, and I knew there was an opportunity to grow with every investigation of them. Their first declaration was that this was Lyme again. I spoke to Dr. Gruber and we reinstated a few supportive supplements and I tightened up my diet. It was interesting to notice how easy it was to be a slacker when it came to diet. It did not escape my notice that as soon as I began to take the supplements I immediately had an experience of kindness. Within a couple of weeks I was beginning to feel normal again.

I started to realize that during the last year I had laboriously lain down a fresh foundation for wellness. The cement hadn't had time to set when I began dancing all over it in my enthusiasm. The truly responsible thing for me to do was to walk softly and allow the foundation to set over time. As it turned out, the time required was almost a year. It was the year of living gently.

It was more than twelve months later that I experienced another round of symptoms. I noticed that despite it being so much further away from that last year of illness, my mind still had a knee jerk reaction and panicked about a relapse of Lyme disease. It was revealed that I was having a candida flare-up, and in response to Dr. Gruber's questions, it became apparent that a current long-term project was adding a great deal of stress to my life, robbing me of sleep and diminishing my appetite. Addressing those lifestyle issues, along with a couple of homeopathic remedies, set me back on track very promptly. That was the last time my thoughts provoked worry about a Lyme relapse.

More recently I had two days of feeling quite unwell with a noticeable fever. When I felt well again I sent an excited message to Dr. Gruber celebrating my body's ability to produce a fever. Through the years of dealing with Lyme, my body would ache as though my temperature was raging. However, mostly it read slightly below normal. He responded with a hearty, "Congratulations!" And then we texted smiley emoticons to each other in a silly but delightful moment of joy. I was not only celebrating the response of a healthy immune system, I had severed ties with Lyme.

CHAPTER 14
The Arrival of Teachers

Something I realized in the knowing of 'I am' was that there is an automatic expression of sharing. I only had good news anyway. I couldn't help but notice that although there were thousands of people dealing with chronic illness, I experienced them as whole and complete. What a pleasure! The very nature of love is to love and embrace, and there are undoubtedly infinite ways to express love. One such way for me was creating opportunities in the community, not to share stories about the suffering or the deep struggles of dealing with illness, but uplifting explorations into the truth of who we are, acknowledging the challenges at hand but then using them as an access to self-discovery. The Lymethriving Facebook page was born and my friend Lisa and I began hosting free teleconference calls. In time these activities expanded to include retreats. It was as though they created themselves.

For many years I had been drawn to the exploration of spirituality. I didn't consider myself a student of anything in particular, it was just an ever-present curiosity that, when tended to, felt nourishing. I had flown through the pages of more books than I could remember, by a variety of authors. Mostly I couldn't remember their names or the titles of the books, although an occasional one would stand out. It was interesting to read about people's past life regressions, appearances of spirit guides, angelic realms and metaphysical explorations. During those years I was fortunate to have a mentor, Tullia, who, knowing a lot about where I was in my life's journey, made recommendations that she felt would be helpful and revealing. I had no attachment to any particular tradition or philosophy, finding that gleaning what resonated with me out of each particular book was quite satisfying.

A few months into wellness, someone suggested I might enjoy listening to the teachings of Gangaji. I'd never heard of her and so asked for the spelling of her name. "Look for her on YouTube," I was told. The weeks that followed were like a celebration of recognition. I watched hours upon hours of videos, saturating myself in the soothing sound of her voice and her deep clarity. She was giving language to the ineffable. Gangaji's use of vocabulary sang in harmony with my own and her investigations into the nature of who we are facilitated a deepening of my own understandings. She was the first teacher who appeared in my new life.

About a year later a Facebook friend sent me an email with a link to a video. All she had written was (I paraphrase), "In reading your postings I feel you will enjoy this teacher." It was a ten-minute video of Rupert Spira interacting with one of his retreat participants. The woman was struggling with her response to Lyme and her thoughts about ending her life. It was beautiful! In a gentle conversation he assisted her, in revealing to herself, what I had come to realize but had never been able to articulate so clearly. It pointed to true healing, which has nothing to do with the body being cured of illness. And so again, I immersed myself in hours of videos. Rupert's unassuming manner, his British accent and a remarkable clarity made it that much more enjoyable. A second teacher had appeared.

As time went on a few more teachers became known to me. What I like about all of them, and why I sometimes mention them to other people, is that just as I had realized that no teacher or teaching was required for waking up, these teachers did not stand in a position of sharing information to be remembered and followed. They always pointed back to the person, inviting (and not requiring) them to discover for themselves what was already present and always had been. They are inviting them to explore their own experience. The gift they offer is love. In an embrace without judgment, they encourage and offer company during self-investigation, and they recognize that everyone is just the same.

It was with absolute joy that I participated in two retreats with Rupert. In some ways it was not what I had expected. My past experience had been self-development courses that covered multiple days, each of which was delivered inside of a rigid structure and set of rules. The courses had been extraordinary in the tools they provided, and I continue to enjoy the benefits, most especially as I applied them in distinguishing disempowering thoughts and beliefs during my last year of illness. So there I was, on retreat. There were no rules. All I knew was the start time of each of the two daily sessions and our meals. Everyone was in their seats on time, there were no side conversations, and any topic could be brought up for discussion. What struck me most was the absence of stories being shared. The participants were interested only in uncovering what was beneath their circumstances. Rupert's clarity went far beyond what I had enjoyed in the videos, and my understanding deepened. We spent the week in a relaxed and easy way, enjoying meals together, long conversations, lots of laughter and tears, walks in nature and times of silence, and Rupert was just one of us.

At the beginning of my first year of wellness I wondered if the experience of life could possibly get better, or if perhaps the majority of my life's chapters were complete. As I left my first Rupert retreat, I knew experientially that in fact, not only was it possible for life to continue to deepen in its richness, but that I was not yet complete with the *first* chapter in my life. I didn't know what else there was, but standing comfortably in not knowing was exquisite.

CHAPTER 15
The Slow Road to Cognitive Repair

Cognitive dysfunction was an especially interesting and challenging part of the Lyme experience. It was also one of the few symptoms that evoked some immediate fear as I became aware of the disconnect in my brain's function. My initial realization of this dysfunction was when I repeatedly found I was forgetting to do things I'd promised to do. Nothing major, just a lot of little small things. I'd write a to-do-list to help myself remember something, and at the end of the day Dennis would ask if I'd done them and I would find I had little to no recollection of the prior discussion, let alone the fact that I'd written myself a note.

As it escalated I had experiences of finding myself driving in my car with absolutely no idea of where I was heading to or where I was driving from. But by that point I had begun to notice I was aware of this happening, meaning I was aware that I was driving and also aware that I was forgetting something. It was interesting to me that I had crystal clarity about the fact that I was in a moment of memory loss, and would wonder what it was that was aware of this, because in the moment my brain was blank.

In the last months of illness my cognitive function seemed normal. I was no longer having memory lapses or speech issues, but I was aware that a particular function still seemed disrupted. Without concern or worry about it, I went on with life. In December of 2011 I was closing out my small business financials in preparation for tax filings. As was my usual routine, I handed my set of financials to Dennis for review and he did what he normally did: prompted me to pass through a couple of closing entries to correct and complete them for the year-end. I promptly burst into tears. In complete surprise he asked what was wrong; I explained that I had no idea how to do that. He stared at me, almost in disbelief, and said, "But you've done these types of entries hundreds of times over the years!" I explained that as soon as he said to create the journal entries, all I could see was a blank sheet of white paper. It seemed as though I had absolutely no access to this old knowledge. And so he gave me the instructions like a paint by numbers project, and I followed each word and letter carefully and closed out my books. I had no idea what I was doing but I knew I could follow the instructions. There was something about numbers that wasn't working properly. I could perform normal mathematical functions but in a context where the numbers related to each other there was a void. After that incident I made peace with this leftover symptom, knowing that I might just need assistance going forward. I was fine with that.

Almost two years into wellness I got involved with a very large financial project that was surrounded by a great deal of urgency. It required pulling together years' worth of financial information to create a clean set of financials. I was quite happy to offer my support by taking this on and looked forward to completing it, but I came up against my brain's dysfunction. As I sat in front of my computer, plugging away, I had the repeated experience of my brain feeling as though it was about to short circuit and explode. I didn't pay too much attention to the source of it, I just knew that I had to walk away and take a break. But with the urgency of a deadline I'd soon be back at my desk. About a week into the work I noticed that these episodes were lessening in their frequency, and then one day I had a sudden experience of ease. It was as though my brain had been straining against a barrier and the barrier had suddenly broken. There was immense flow in my thinking process and the mental image of these numbers and how they related to one another began to come into focus. Only then did I realize that the neural pathways that had been disrupted during my illness were now repairing. It felt as though a broken bridge had been repaired and a clear path across a river was now available.

Truly discovering what is possible without any requirement for the discovery is like an amazing surprise party. Where some say healing is not possible, anything is possible. I loved being able to share this slow road to repair with others, to offer this unexpected gift of healing as a beacon of hope in their own unique journey toward wellness.

It was around this time that I read a book by Anita Moorjani called *Dying to Be Me*. After fighting cancer for almost four years, and now with tumors throughout her body, Anita's organs began to fail and she slipped into a coma. Her family was summoned to her side to be with her as she died. During her coma she had an extraordinary near-death experience during which she realized her inherent worth and uncovered the actual cause of her disease - living fearfully. Upon regaining consciousness, Anita improved so rapidly that she was released from the hospital within weeks, without a trace of cancer in her body. Needless to say she became the object of intense scientific study and an inspirational teacher.

Complete and spontaneous healing is what's possible. It is unusual, but it remains possible. Most of us seem to go through a process of healing, but that healing occurs inside the possibility of complete and spontaneous healing. It supports us in various ways to believe we will be well again, and it supports us to believe in our methods of treating our bodies. But what is more powerful is letting go of our attachment to the belief, and simply being open to what's possible. This is aligning with the truth of who we are, and no matter how slow the road to repair, something is possible beyond that which we can imagine.

CHAPTER 16
The Eye of The Needle

There was a continuation of contemplating the nature of experience and the intricacies of life. I was becoming more aware of the non-dual nature of truth. The 'eye of the needle' process had started with noticing what I wasn't, and had evolved into knowing what I am. But there was still some sense of duality with which I was engaged.

After the first retreat with Rupert I floated peacefully through the weeks that followed, in tearful awe of the beauty that is. The ever-familiar trails that I strolled with the dogs revealed gifts that I had been overlooking. Most particularly I was struck by how sunbeams slipped between the leaves of the trees, ever so gently resting on the branches and tree trunks. I could feel the softness of the touch of the light, and it moved me. But over time, as is the human thing to do, I began listening to the commentary in my mind, to a question that it kept posing. And so my mind busied itself trying to find an answer and I revisited Monkey Mind Land.

My mind was grappling with 'knowing' that all objects are perceived in three dimensional space by a finite mind that itself arises in one dimensional time, and was left asking the question, "Does that mean that the universe is finite?" Disappointingly it kept coming up with a yes. I couldn't remember a time in my life when I didn't relish getting lost in a starry night sky, loving the experience of contemplating its endlessness, so for me, a finite universe was an unsettling thought.

I got myself onto a webinar with Rupert to explore this question in the hopes of settling the disturbance of my thoughts. Being led back into my own experience of awareness, he kept asking me questions until that moment that I had my own answer in the experience of knowing it myself. Infinite awareness or consciousness (our true Self) is expressed into our 'reality' as mind and matter in the four dimensions of time and space. The nature of awareness is unbounded, open, non-resistant, all encompassing, infinite love. What we are experiencing as a universe (through seeing, hearing, tasting, touching, smelling, perceiving, feeling, and thinking) is the expression of infinite awareness or consciousness into a time/space reality. So anything and everything in our experience is a knowing of the awareness that is, and that awareness is eternal.

It had been easier to know the Oneness that we are when I looked at people. Somehow it had been clear that the source of me was the one same source for every person on the planet. The one great "I" with billions of different expressions as other people. But my mind had resisted that sameness with objects.

Somehow in that brief webinar conversation, I finally came to know the entire universe as a perception of the expression of infinite awareness as matter. It did not matter that it was being perceived through a finite mind because the source of the mind was awareness too. It was instantly clear that everyTHING is also OF the I that I am and that we each are. The beauty of this is so exquisite it is beyond the description of words. It is so much more beautiful than simply being matter that goes on indefinitely, and certainly beyond the mind's ability to know.

In that moment all things were leveled to sameness. It was not that things I held on a higher level came down to a same lower level, it was all things being raised to an exquisite sameness, all in and of consciousness. I was present to that exquisiteness in the computer I was looking at, the trees outside the window and my own Self. The intimacy with all of life was closer than my heart beat and yet completely impersonal to the me I think of as a separate self. With no words to adequately express my gratitude for Rupert's guidance or to convey the revelation, I simply shared through my tears that I felt it in my heart. And as is Rupert's way, he smiled humbly and went on to the next person's question.

After recognizing what I wasn't, I had begun, through the illness experience, re-identifying with that which I truly am, the awareness of 'I am.' In fully letting go I had passed through the eye of the needle completely only now to discover that all I had recognized to not be me was actually still there and still OF the I that I am. The furthest reaches of the universe were intimately one with me. And in all humbleness I knew that I had finally completed Chapter One of my life.

The investigations and inquiries continue. At this particular point in my journey I notice a couple of things that are shifting. I more readily allow myself to simply experience the moment. I'm aware of my thoughts about those moments but my interest is primarily on the actual experience itself. The more familiar I become with the mechanisms of how I am being human, the greater my level of compassion for others as I recognize myself in them. There are extended periods of time where peace is so profoundly present that I have a sense of not being attached to anything, including being alive, and it is glorious. However, I sometimes find myself humbled when I recognize that there will not be a time when a hidden anchor or long held belief can't be revealed.

We make it so complicated, although I don't think it's a mistake that we do. The simplicity of simply being aware of being aware is easily overlooked as we are distracted with our thoughts, feelings and perceptions and identifying ourselves with a separate self. To be fully present in the now is the greatest gift we can give ourselves. It takes no effort and no knowledge and no special practice, although any of those three might be useful along the way. And while my mind has named different people and beloved animals as teachers, the greatest teacher of all is the experience of life itself, begging to be experienced in all its rawness. The best of our human teachers do not actually teach, they just point us in the direction of home...consciousness. We can give ourselves freely to all that life has to offer, knowing all along that we are living an illusionary story in which we are one of the characters.

Someone once shared an analogy that is now a favorite of mine. Consciousness or awareness, the 'I' that we are, is like the screen on which a movie is played. Regardless of how the story plays out on the screen, the screen remains the same at all times, unchanged and un-impacted by any drama that plays out on it. We might recognize a character in the story as our body/mind, and we fully relate and are aware of all his or her experiences. But not one experience is part of our actual identity. We are simply the screen, resisting no part of the story being played on it. The screen can exist without the story, but the story requires the screen to exist. It is profoundly moving to know that who we truly are resists nothing. It is fully allowing in love and war, kindness and hatefulness. This is unconditional love. This is who we are.

CHAPTER 17
What is Your First Step, and Why?

In completing my book it seems appropriate to address the three questions I am asked most frequently.

"Where do I begin and what are the steps I should follow?"

To start with let me just assure you that there is no script to follow and you can't get it wrong. All we have is this very moment, and in this moment we already have all we need. It's just a matter of removing each layer that inhibits the light of ourselves from shining forth. Whatever is most active in your awareness right now is indicating your starting point. If there are several things, just pick one. For me it was resisting that I was chronically ill. As you address each step of your own journey, you might need to remind yourself that sometimes we are faced with similar issues repeatedly, not because we have failed, but because sometimes we are simply ready to take an old lesson to a new level of understanding. As we resolve something, a clearing is revealed in which our next step becomes apparent. This often feels like one step forward, two steps back.

Consider that when we find ourselves unwell, our foundation is uneven, and the symptoms of this are reflected like the cracks in the walls of a building. In all appropriateness, we tend to the symptoms to make ourselves more comfortable, and hopefully at the same time, work at re-leveling the foundation so that the sealed up cracks in the walls do not reopen.

But re-leveling a foundation takes time and effort. As we address one part of the foundation it has an impact on the whole structure as it resettles and it might produce a new crack in the wall. This is the experience of two steps back.

It is normal to find ourselves resisting the next step when we have just relieved ourselves of an emotional burden, but even our reaction to the next step can reveal something to us about ourselves. Be kind to yourself and trust that you are not stuck in the dead end of a maze, you have simply reached a sharp turn in the bend of a labyrinth and what lies ahead is simply out of view. I promise that no matter what you discover about yourself, it is worthy of love.

"What practices did you follow?"

While I have dabbled here and there in yoga and meditation, I have not had a regular practice in either. The only day in and day out practice I followed was to be aware of my thoughts. I didn't try to change them, I just began to notice them until it was an established practice. From there I began to notice the nature of my thoughts and how often I believed them to be the truth, and where my thoughts were interpreting life and all its circumstances and providing opinions that masqueraded as conclusions. I have a sense that incorporating a new practice(s) into my life, along with this ongoing thought awareness, will be very beneficial. The time is drawing closer.

"Will I get well if I do my internal work?"

I am also frequently asked about the purpose or benefits of doing our 'internal work' and if it will make a body heal from illness. I say discover who you are simply because it's the truth. Know yourself as whole and complete, simply because it's the truth. Know yourself as peace, simply because it's the truth. And, from that knowing, tend to the body in whatever way feels right for you. When you are identified with your true Self, you will offer a vibration that is aligned with wellbeing and wellness. It will support your body in healing. It can't not help. Whether you recover fully or not, whether your path to wellness is long or short, you will enjoy a richness in life that nothing can diminish.

CHAPTER 18
How Can I Support You?

Please visit www.lymethriving.com for information on the following:

FREE TELECONFERENCES: Recordings of all our previous teleconferences that address the spiritual and emotional component of chronic illness, and listings of any upcoming scheduled calls. There are also plenty of recordings of teleconferences with guest speakers who offer their particular expertise in addressing the physical aspect of Lyme and other tick-borne illnesses.

RETREATS: Listings of upcoming retreats and speaking events for anyone dealing with chronic illnesses. The retreats and meetings do not address the treatment of illness, but focus on using the experience of illness to realize the truth of who we are, supporting us to bring peace forward into our current circumstances.

RECOMMENDED READING LIST: A list of some of my personal favorites.

GUIDED MEDITATIONS: YouTube videos with teachers masterful in leading us into self-discovery.

NEWSLETTERS: Sign up to receive newsletters about upcoming events and offerings.

Acknowledgements

My team of healthcare professionals and healing practitioners: Gary Gruber, ND, Chris Bonnemort, Dr. Mitchell Gordon, Dr. Lawrence Stern, Cynthia Farina and Bernadette Bloom. Thank you for your knowledge, wisdom and caring.

To my dear friends Phyllie Conroy and Pamela Yates, who's homes I visited every couple of weeks throughout my illness, where I curled up in blankets, slept through TV movies, sipped wine and received the unconditional support of deep friendship. Thank you seems so inadequate.

The pre-editor editors of this book: Mum, Sarah Ruminski, Samantha Rush, Pamela Yates, Phyllie Conroy.........I am so grateful for your willingness to take the time to read this story and offer feedback and edits as it developed.

My gratitude to Amy B. Scher who generously offers guidance and support in all my projects and especially this one.

My appreciation to my editor Dr. Michael of FirstEditing.com for prompt and clear editing suggestions.

Thank you Lisa Hilton for partnering with me as we launched the teleconferences. Your years of dedication to supporting others in the Lyme community is a testament to your generous heart.

Love and gratitude to Fran Swart and Jenna Wright who have teamed up with me to co-host retreats. Your special gifts of service and support are immeasurable.

To the Lyme disease and tick-borne illness community, I feel blessed to be a part of this family. Your friendship and company through my darkest days will never be forgotten. Thank you for sharing yourselves with me and allowing me to share myself with you. It is truly a privilege to call you friends and to know you as my chosen family. It is my hope that in some way I am able to support you and other chronic illness patients into the realization of peace, regardless of what you are experiencing in illness. A heartfelt acknowledgment to all the movers and shakers who continue to stand for transforming the way chronic Lyme and co-infections are dealt with in the political, medical and insurance arenas.

CPSIA information can be obtained
at www.ICGtesting.com
Printed in the USA
BVOW06s0323200817
492488BV00006B/15/P

9 781495 182334